The Complete Mediterranean Delicacies Dishes

Fit and Healthy on a Budget Recipes to Burn Fat

Alison Russell

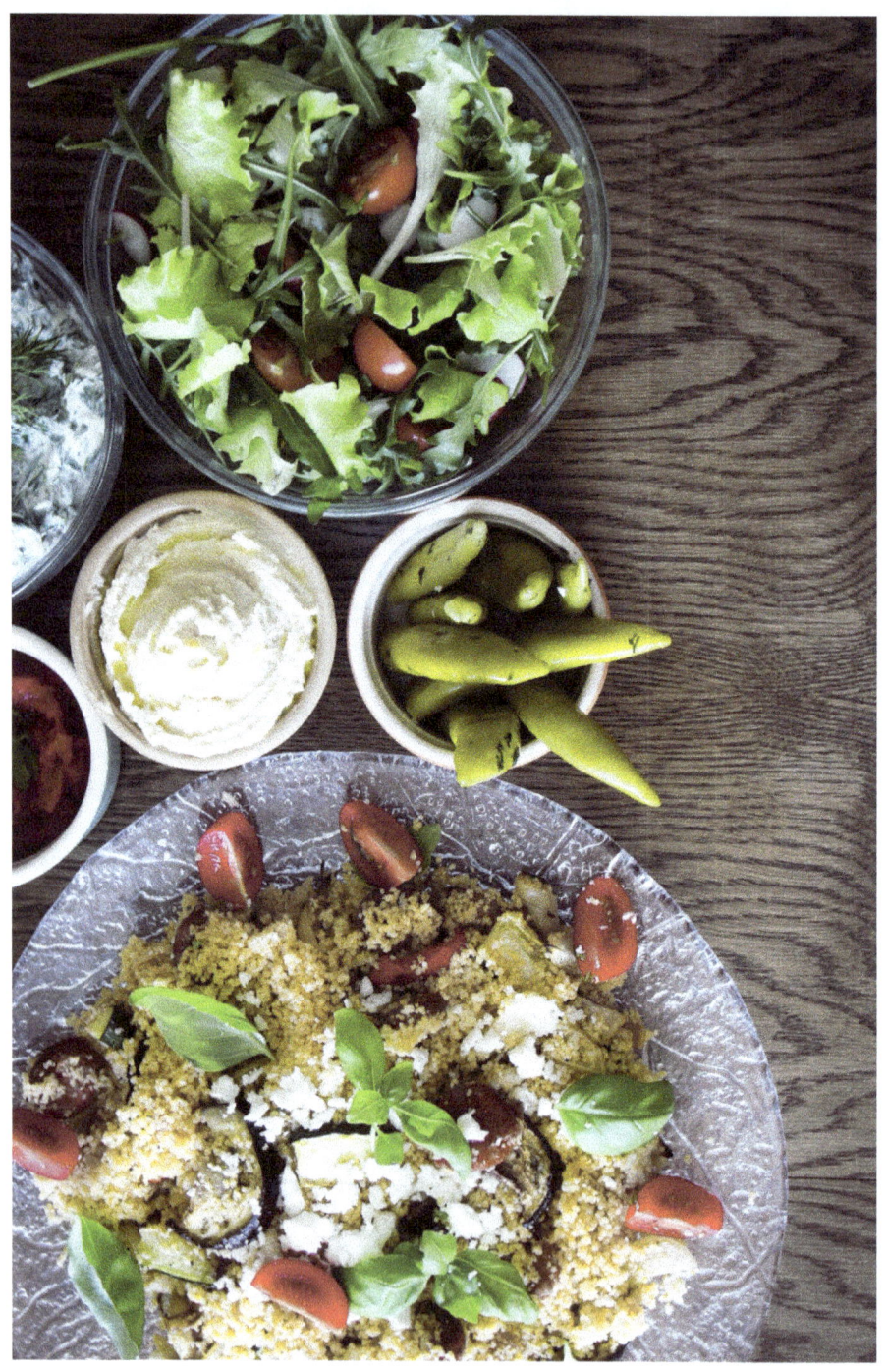

© **Copyright 2020 - All rights reserved.**

The content contained within this book may not be reproduced, duplicated or transmitted without direct written permission from the author or the publisher.

Under no circumstances will any blame or legal responsibility be held against the publisher, or author, for any damages, reparation, or monetary loss due to the information contained within this book. Either directly or indirectly.

Legal Notice:

This book is copyright protected. This book is only for personal use. You cannot amend, distribute, sell, use, quote or paraphrase any part, or the content within this book, without the consent of the author or publisher.

Disclaimer Notice:

Please note the information contained within this document is for educational and entertainment purposes only. All effort has been executed to present accurate, up to date, and reliable, complete information. No warranties of any kind are declared or implied. Readers acknowledge that the author is not engaging in the rendering of legal, financial, medical or professional advice. The content within this book has been derived from various sources. Please consult a licensed professional before attempting any techniques outlined in this book.

By reading this document, the reader agrees that under no circumstances is the author responsible for any losses, direct or indirect, which are incurred as a result of the use of information contained within this document, including, but not limited to, — errors, omissions, or inaccuracies.

Table of contents

Beans, Grains, and Pastas 8

    Spinach and Ricotta Stuffed Pasta Shells 9

    Chili Halloumi Cheese with Rice 12

    Grana Padano Risotto 13

    Turkey and Bell Pepper Tortiglioni 15

    Carrot Risoni 17

    Roasted Butternut Squash and Rice 19

    Pesto Arborio Rice and Veggie Bowls 21

    Rice and Bean Stuffed Zucchini 24

Vegetable Mains 26

    Brussels Sprouts Linguine 27

    Beet and Watercress Salad 30

    Garlicky Broccoli Rabe 32

    Sautéed Cabbage with Parsley 34

    Braised Cauliflower with White Wine 37

    Cauliflower Steaks with Arugula 39

    Parmesan Stuffed Zucchini Boats 41

    Baby Kale and Cabbage Salad 44

    Grilled Romaine Lettuce 46

    Mini Crustless Spinach Quiches 47

Butternut Noodles with Mushrooms 49

Potato Tortilla with Leeks and Mushrooms 51

Mushrooms Ragu with Cheesy Polenta 54

Veggie Rice Bowls with Pesto Sauce 56

Roasted Cauliflower and Carrots 58

Saut é ed Spinach and Leeks 60

Zoodles with Beet Pesto 61

Fried Eggplant Rolls 63

Garlicky Zucchini Cubes with Mint 65

Zucchini and Artichokes Bowl with Farro 67

Zucchini Fritters 69

Fish and Seafood 71

Mussels with Onions 72

Cod Curry 74

Shrimps with Northern Beans 76

Shrimp and Potato Curry 78

Sardines and Plum Tomato Curry 80

Salmon and Mushroom Hash with Pesto 81

Spiced Citrus Sole 84

Asian-Inspired Tuna Lettuce Wraps 86

Crispy Tilapia with Mango Salsa 87

Mediterranean Grilled Sea Bass 89

Braised Branzino with Wine Sauce 91

Peppercorn-Seared Tuna Steaks 93

Canned Sardine Donburi (Rice Bowl) 94

Baked Halibut Steaks with Vegetables 96

Spicy Haddock Stew 98

Orange Flavored Scallops 100

Garlic Skillet Salmon 102

Fruits and Desserts 104

Chocolate, Almond, and Cherry Clusters 105

Chocolate and Avocado Mousse 106

Coconut Blueberries with Brown Rice 107

Blueberry and Oat Crisp 108

Beans, Grains, and Pastas

Spinach and Ricotta Stuffed Pasta Shells

Prep time: 15 minutes | Cook time: 35 minutes | Serves 6

- 2 cups onion, chopped
- 1 cup carrot, chopped
- 3 garlic cloves, minced
- 3½ tablespoons olive oil,
- 1 (28-ounce / 794-g) canned tomatoes, crushed
- 12 ounces (340 g) conchiglie pasta
- 1 tablespoon olive oil
- 2 cups ricotta cheese, crumbled
- 1½ cups feta cheese, crumbled
- 2 cups spinach, chopped
- ¾ cup grated Pecorino Romano cheese
- 2 tablespoons chopped fresh chives
- 1 tablespoon chopped fresh dill
- Salt and ground black pepper to taste
- 1 cup shredded Cheddar cheese

1. Warm olive oil on Sauté. Add onion, carrot, and garlic, and cook for 5 minutes until tender. Stir in tomatoes and cook for another 10 minutes. Remove to a bowl and set aside.
2. Wipe the pot with a damp cloth, add pasta and cover with enough water. Seal the lid and cook

for 5 minutes on High Pressure. Do a quick release and drain the pasta. Lightly Grease olive oil to a baking sheet.
3. In a bowl, combine feta and ricotta cheese. Add spinach, Pecorino Romano cheese, dill, and chives, and stir well. Adjust the seasonings. Using a spoon, fill the shells with the mixture.
4. Spread 4 cups tomato sauce on the baking sheet. Place the stuffed shells over with seam-sides down and sprinkle Cheddar cheese atop. Use aluminum foil to the cover the baking dish.
5. Pour 1 cup of water in the pot of the Pressure cooker and insert the trivet. Lower the baking dish onto the trivet. Seal the lid, and cook for 15 minutes on High Pressure. Do a quick pressure release. Take away the foil. Place the stuffed shells to serving plates and top with tomato sauce before serving.

Per Serving

calories: 730 | fat: 41.5g | protein: 30.0g | carbs: 62.7g | fiber: 10.6g | sodium: 966mg

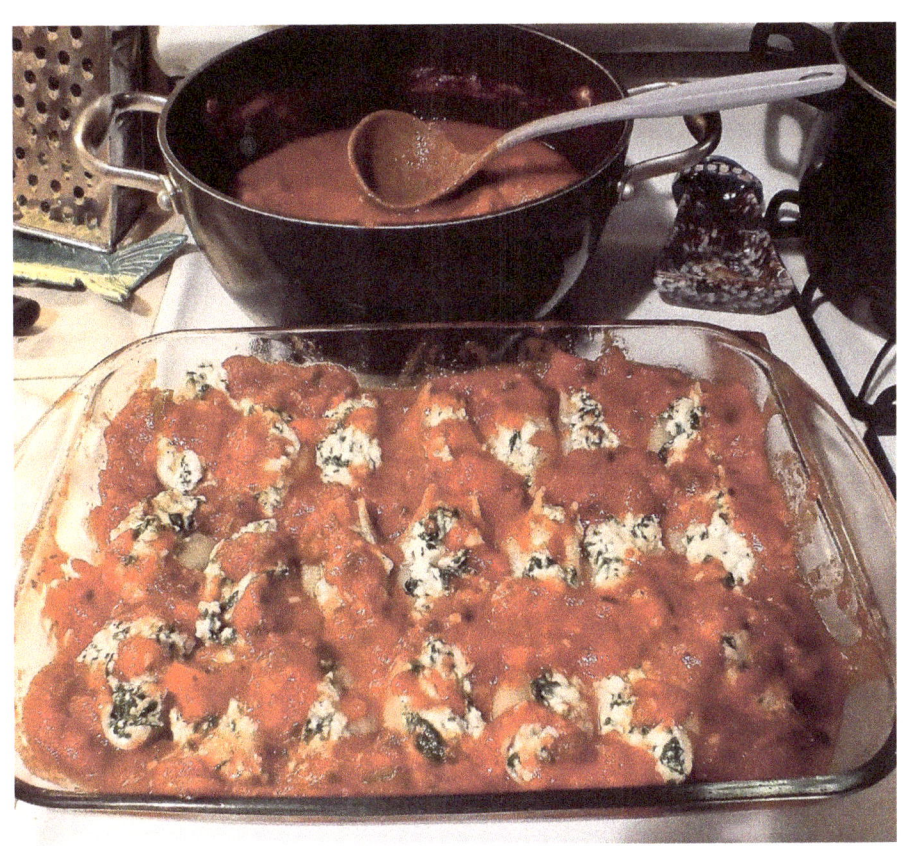

Chili Halloumi Cheese with Rice

Prep time: 10 minutes | Cook time: 8 minutes | Serves 6

- 2 cups water
- 2 tablespoons brown sugar
- 2 tablespoons rice vinegar
- 1 tablespoon sweet chili sauce
- 1 tablespoon olive oil
- 1 teaspoon fresh minced garlic
- 20 ounces (567 g) Halloumi cheese, cubed
- 1 cup rice
- ¼ cup chopped fresh chives, for garnish

1. Heat the oil on Sauté and fry the halloumi for 5 minutes until golden brown. Set aside.
2. To the pot, add water, garlic, olive oil, vinegar, sugar, soy sauce, and chili sauce and mix well until smooth. Stir in rice noodles. Seal the lid and cook on High Pressure for 3 minutes. Release the pressure quickly. Split the rice between bowls. Top with fried halloumi and sprinkle with fresh chives before serving.

Per Serving

calories: 534 | fat: 34.3g | protein: 24.9g | carbs: 30.1g | fiber: 1.0g | sodium: 652mg

Grana Padano Risotto

Prep time: 10 minutes | Cook time: 23 minutes | Serves 6

- 1 tablespoon olive oil
- 1 white onion, chopped
- 2 cups Carnaroli rice, rinsed
- ¼ cup dry white wine
- 4 cups chicken stock
- 1 teaspoon salt
- ½ teaspoon ground white pepper
- 2 tablespoons Grana padano cheese, grated
- ¼ tablespoon Grana padano cheese, flakes

1. Warm oil on Sauté. Stir-fry onion for 3 minutes until soft and translucent. Add rice and cook for 5 minutes stirring occasionally.
2. Pour wine into the pot to deglaze, scrape away any browned bits of food from the pan.
3. Stir in stock, pepper, and salt to the pot. Seal the lid, press Rice and cook on High Pressure for 15 minutes. Release the pressure quickly.
4. Sprinkle with grated Parmesan cheese and stir well. Top with flaked cheese for garnish before serving.

Per Serving

calories: 307 | fat: 6.0g | protein: 8.2g | carbs: 53.2g | fiber: 2.1g | sodium: 945mg

Turkey and Bell Pepper Tortiglioni

Prep time: 20 minutes | Cook time: 10 minutes | Serves 6

2 teaspoons chili powder

1 teaspoon salt

1 teaspoon cumin

1 teaspoon onion powder

1 teaspoon garlic powder

½ teaspoon thyme

1½ pounds (680 g) turkey breast, cut into strips

1 tablespoon olive oil

1 red onion, cut into wedges

4 garlic cloves, minced

3 cups chicken broth

1 cup salsa

1 pound (454 g) tortiglioni

1 red bell pepper, chopped diagonally

1 yellow bell pepper, chopped diagonally

1 green bell pepper, chopped diagonally

1 cup shredded Gouda cheese

½ cup sour cream

½ cup chopped parsley

1. In a bowl, mix chili powder, cumin, garlic powder, onion powder, salt, and oregano. Reserve 1 teaspoon of seasoning. Coat turkey with the remaining seasoning.

2. Warm oil on Sauté. Add turkey strips and sauté for 4 to 5 minutes until browned. Place the turkey in a bowl. Sauté the onion and garlic for 1 minute in the cooker until soft. Press Cancel.
3. Mix in salsa, broth, and scrape the bottom of any brown bits. Into the broth mixture, stir in tortiglioni pasta and cover with bell peppers and chicken.
4. Seal the lid and cook for 5 minutes on High Pressure. Do a quick Pressure release.
5. Open the lid and sprinkle with shredded gouda cheese and reserved seasoning, and stir well. Divide into plates and top with sour cream. Add parsley for garnishing and serve.

Per Serving

calories: 646 | fat: 21.7g | protein: 41.1g | carbs: 72.9g | fiber: 11.1g | sodium: 1331mg

Carrot Risoni

Prep time: 5 minutes | Cook time: 11 minutes | Serves 6

- 1 cup orzo, rinsed
- 2 cups water
- 2 carrots, cut into sticks
- 1 large onion, chopped
- 2 tablespoons olive oil
- Salt, to taste
- Fresh cilantro, chopped, for garnish

1. Heat oil on Sauté. Add onion and carrots and stir-fry for about 10 minutes until tender and crispy. Remove to a plate and set aside. Add water, salt and orzo in the instant pot.
2. Seal the lid and cook on High Pressure for 1 minute. Do a quick release. Fluff the cooked orzo with a fork. Transfer to a serving plate and top with the carrots and onion. Serve scattered with cilantro.

Per Serving

calories: 121 | fat: 4.9g | protein: 1.7g | carbs: 18.1g | fiber: 2.9g | sodium: 17mg

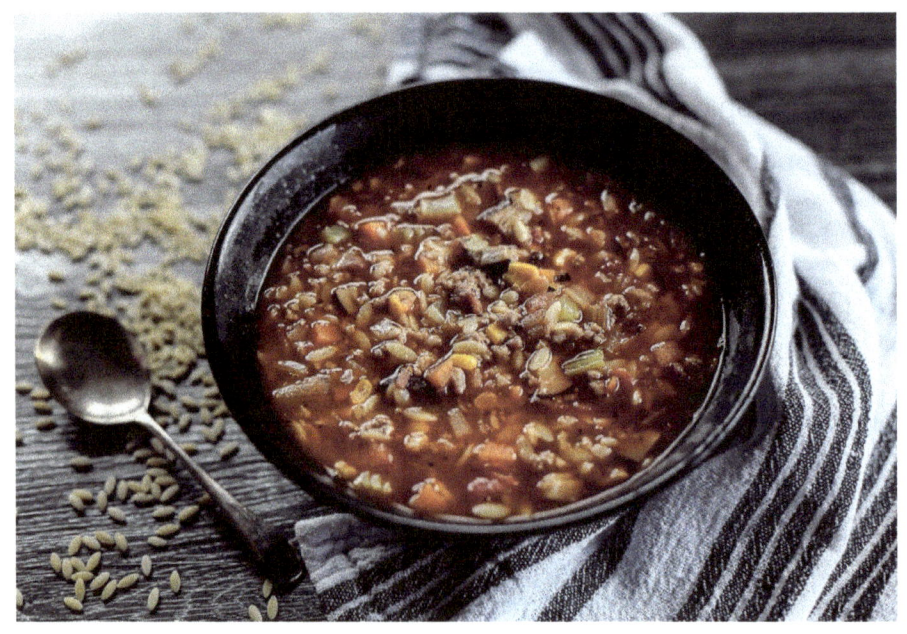

Roasted Butternut Squash and Rice

Prep time: 15 minutes | Cook time: 15 minutes | Serves 4

- ½ cup water
- 2 cups vegetable broth
- 1 small butternut squash, peeled and sliced
- 2 tablespoons olive oil, divided
- 1 teaspoon salt
- 1 teaspoon freshly ground black pepper
- 1 cup feta cheese, cubed
- 1 tablespoon coconut aminos
- 2 teaspoons arrowroot starch
- 1 cup jasmine rice, cooked

1. Pour the rice and broth in the pot and stir to combine. In a bowl, toss butternut squash with 1 tablespoon of olive oil and season with salt and black pepper.
2. In another bowl, mix the remaining olive oil, water and coconut aminos. Toss feta in the mixture, add the arrowroot starch, and toss again to combine well. Transfer to a greased baking dish.

3. Lay a trivet over the rice and place the baking dish on the trivet. Seal the lid and cook on High for 15 minutes. Do a quick pressure release. Fluff the rice with a fork and serve with squash and feta.

Per Serving

calories: 258 | fat: 14.9g | protein: 7.8g | carbs: 23.2g | fiber: 1.2g | sodium: 1180mg

Pesto Arborio Rice and Veggie Bowls

Prep time: 10 minutes | Cook time: 1 minute | Serves 2

1 cup arborio rice, rinsed and drained

2 cups vegetable broth

Salt and black pepper to taste

1 potato, peeled, cubed

1 head broccoli, cut into small florets

1 bunch baby carrots, peeled

¼ cabbage, chopped

2 eggs

¼ cup pesto sauce

Lemon wedges, for serving

1. In the pot, mix broth, pepper, rice and salt. Set trivet to the inner pot on top of rice and add a steamer basket to the top of the trivet. Mix carrots, potato, eggs and broccoli in the steamer basket. Add pepper and salt for seasoning.
2. Seal the lid and cook for 1 minute on High Pressure. Quick release the pressure.
3. Take away the trivet and steamer basket from the pot. Set the eggs in a bowl of ice water. Then peel and halve the eggs. Use a fork to fluff rice. Adjust the seasonings.

4. In two bowls, equally divide rice, broccoli, eggs, carrots, sweet potatoes, and a dollop of pesto. Serve alongside a lemon wedge.

Per Serving

calories: 858 | fat: 24.4g | protein: 26.4g | carbs: 136.2g | fiber: 14.1g | sodium: 985mg

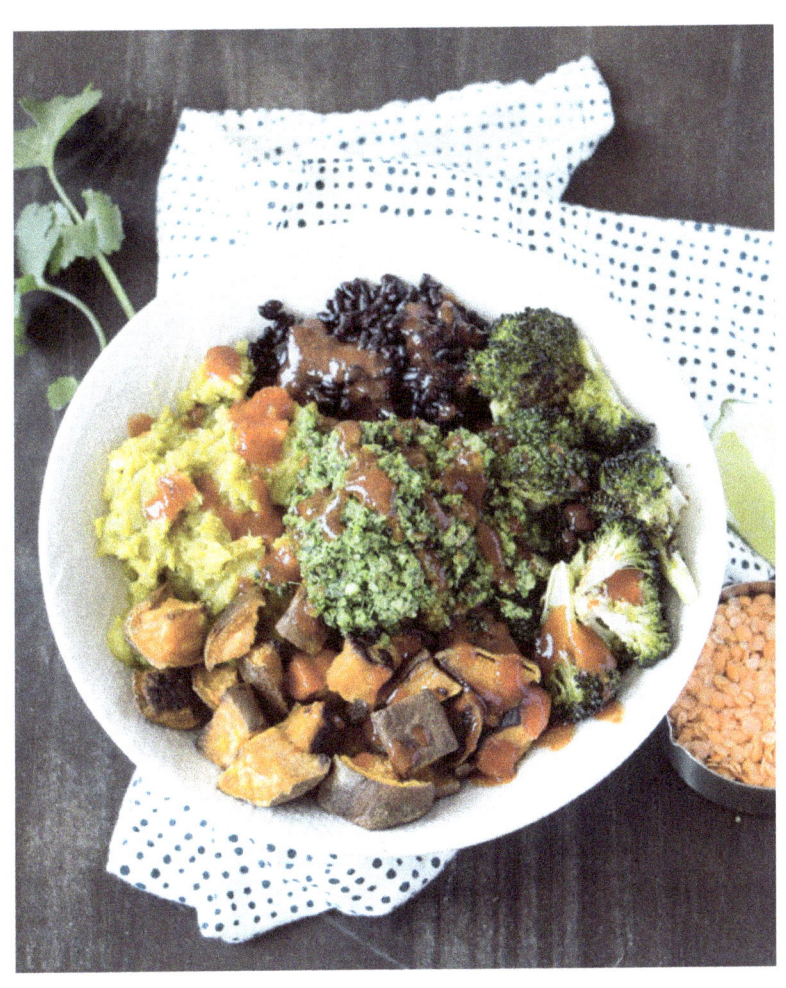

Rice and Bean Stuffed Zucchini

Prep time: 10 minutes | Cook time: 15 minutes | Serves 4

- 2 small zucchinis, halved lengthwise
- ½ cup cooked rice
- ½ cup canned white beans, drained and rinsed
- ½ cup chopped tomatoes
- ½ cup chopped toasted cashew nuts
- ½ cup grated Parmesan cheese
- 1 tablespoon olive oil
- ½ teaspoon salt
- ½ teaspoon freshly ground black pepper

1. Pour 1 cup of water in the instant pot and insert a trivet. Scoop out the pulp of zucchini and chop roughly.
2. In a bowl, mix the zucchini pulp, rice, tomatoes, cashew nuts, ¼ cup of Parmesan, olive oil, salt, and black pepper. Fill the zucchini boats with the mixture, and arrange the stuffed boats in a single layer on the trivet. Seal the lid and cook for 15 minutes on Steam on High. Do a quick release and serve.

Per Serving

calories: 239 | fat: 14.7g | protein: 9.4g | carbs: 19.0g | fiber: 2.6g | sodium: 570mg

Vegetable Mains

Brussels Sprouts Linguine

Prep time: 5 minutes | Cook time: 25 minutes | Serves 4

8 ounces (227 g) whole-wheat linguine

¼ cup plus 2 tablespoons extra-virgin olive oil, divided

1 medium sweet onion, diced

2 to 3 garlic cloves, smashed

8 ounces (227 g) Brussels sprouts, chopped

½ cup chicken stock

¼ cup dry white wine

½ cup shredded Parmesan cheese

1 lemon, quartered

1. Bring a large pot of water to a boil and cook the pasta for about 5 minutes, or until al dente. Drain the pasta and reserve 1 cup of the pasta water. Mix the cooked pasta with 2 tablespoons of the olive oil. Set aside.
2. In a large skillet, heat the remaining ¼ cup of the olive oil over medium heat. Add the onion to the skillet and sauté for about 4 minutes, or until tender. Add the smashed garlic cloves and sauté for 1 minute, or until fragrant.
3. Stir in the Brussels sprouts and cook covered for 10 minutes. Pour in the chicken stock to

prevent burning. Once the Brussels sprouts have wilted and are fork-tender, add white wine and cook for about 5 minutes, or until reduced.
4. Add the pasta to the skillet and add the pasta water as needed.
5. Top with the Parmesan cheese and squeeze the lemon over the dish right before eating.

Per Serving

calories: 502 | fat: 31.0g | protein: 15.0g | carbs: 50.0g | fiber: 9.0g | sodium: 246mg

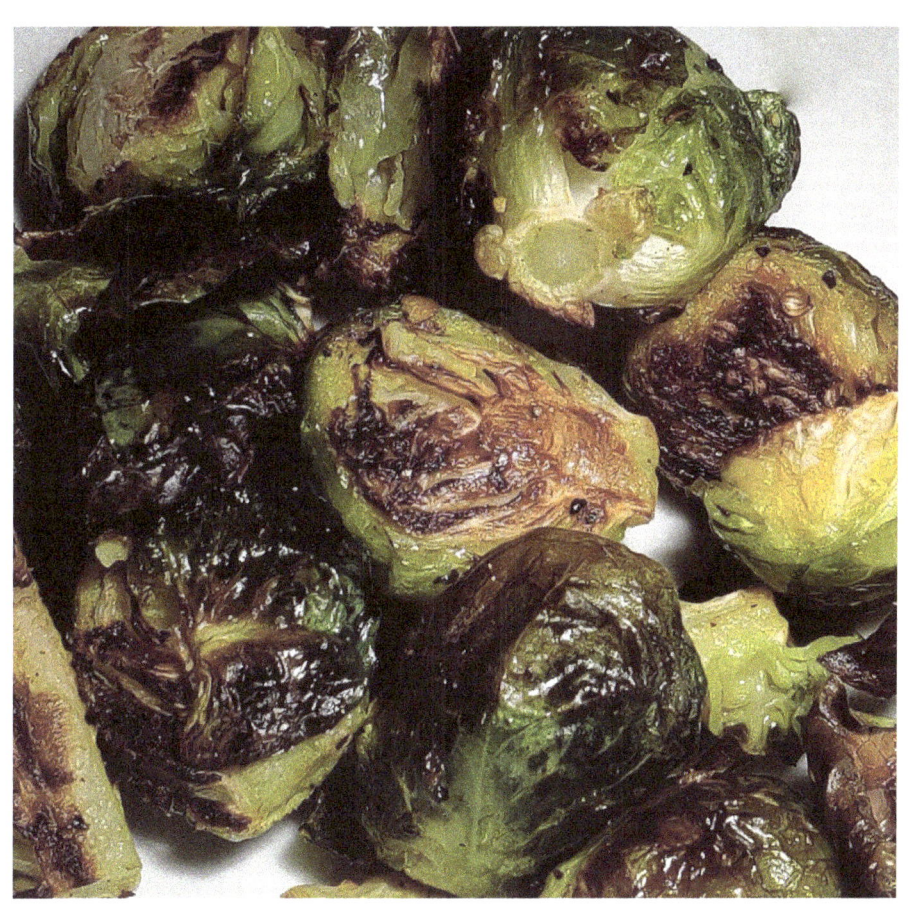

Beet and Watercress Salad

Prep time: 15 minutes | Cook time: 8 minutes | Serves 4

- 2 pounds (907 g) beets, scrubbed, trimmed and cut into ¾-inch pieces
- ½ cup water
- 1 teaspoon caraway seeds
- ½ teaspoon table salt, plus more for seasoning
- 1 cup plain Greek yogurt
- 1 small garlic clove, minced
- 5 ounces (142 g) watercress, torn into bite-size pieces
- 1 tablespoon extra-virgin olive oil, divided, plus more for drizzling
- 1 tablespoon white wine vinegar, divided
- Black pepper, to taste
- 1 teaspoon grated orange zest
- 2 tablespoons orange juice
- ¼ cup coarsely chopped fresh dill
- ¼ cup hazelnuts, toasted, skinned and chopped
- Coarse sea salt, to taste

1. Combine the beets, water, caraway seeds and table salt in the Instant Pot. Set the lid in place. Select the Manual mode and set the cooking time for 8 minutes on High Pressure. When the timer goes off, do a quick pressure release.

2. Carefully open the lid. Using a slotted spoon, transfer the beets to a plate. Set aside to cool slightly.
3. In a small bowl, combine the yogurt, garlic and 3 tablespoons of the beet cooking liquid. In a large bowl, toss the watercress with 2 teaspoons of the oil and 1 teaspoon of the vinegar. Season with table salt and pepper.
4. Spread the yogurt mixture over a serving dish. Arrange the watercress on top of the yogurt mixture, leaving 1-inch border of the yogurt mixture.
5. Add the beets to now-empty large bowl and toss with the orange zest and juice, the remaining 2 teaspoons of the vinegar and the remaining 1 teaspoon of the oil. Season with table salt and pepper.
6. Arrange the beets on top of the watercress mixture. Drizzle with the olive oil and sprinkle with the dill, hazelnuts and sea salt.
7. Serve immediately.

Per Serving

calories: 240 | fat: 15.0g | protein: 9.0g | carbs: 19.0g | fiber: 5.0g | sodium: 440mg

Garlicky Broccoli Rabe

Prep time: 10 minutes | Cook time: 5 to 6 minutes | Serves 4

14 ounces (397 g) broccoli rabe, trimmed and cut into 1-inch pieces

2 teaspoons salt, plus more for seasoning

Black pepper, to taste

2 tablespoons extra-virgin olive oil

3 garlic cloves, minced

¼ teaspoon red pepper flakes

1. Bring 3 quarts water to a boil in a large saucepan. Add the broccoli rabe and 2 teaspoons of the salt to the boiling water and cook for 2 to 3 minutes, or until wilted and tender.
2. Drain the broccoli rabe. Transfer to ice water and let sit until chilled. Drain again and pat dry.
3. In a skillet over medium heat, heat the oil and add the garlic and red pepper flakes. Sauté for about 2 minutes, or until the garlic begins to sizzle.

4. Increase the heat to medium-high. Stir in the broccoli rabe and cook for about 1 minute, or until heated through, stirring constantly. Season with salt and pepper.
5. Serve immediately.

Per Serving

calories: 87 | fat: 7.3g | protein: 3.4g | carbs: 4.0g | fiber: 2.9g | sodium: 1196mg

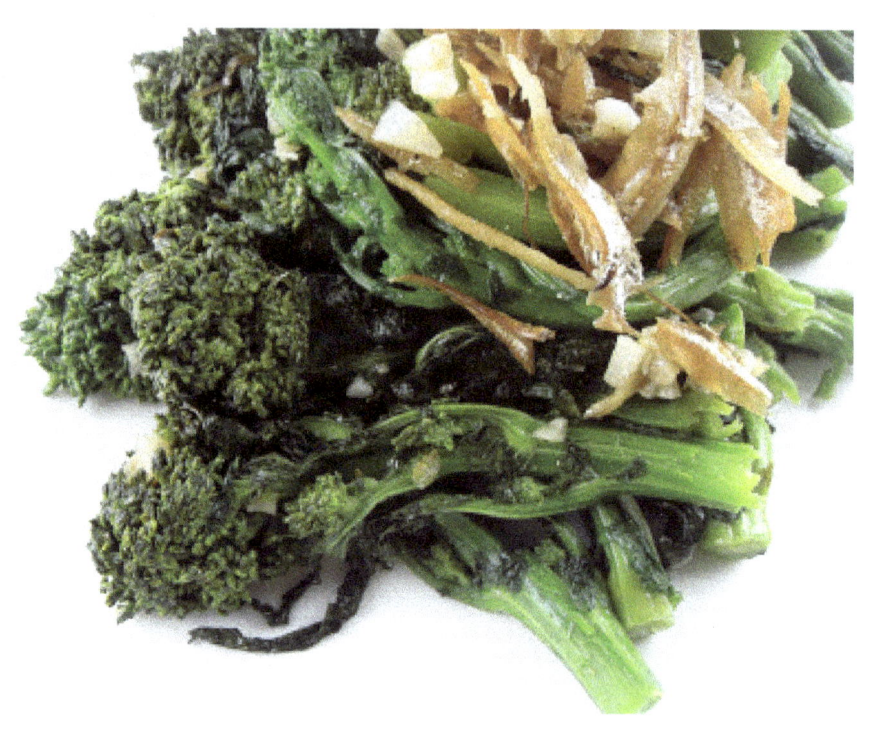

Sautéed Cabbage with Parsley

Prep time: 10 minutes | Cook time: 12 to 14 minutes | Serves 4 to 6

- 1 small head green cabbage (about 1¼ pounds / 567 g), cored and sliced thin
- 2 tablespoons extra-virgin olive oil, divided
- 1 onion, halved and sliced thin
- ¾ teaspoon salt, divided
- ¼ teaspoon black pepper
- ¼ cup chopped fresh parsley
- 1½ teaspoons lemon juice

1. Place the cabbage in a large bowl with cold water. Let sit for 3 minutes. Drain well.
2. Heat 1 tablespoon of the oil in a skillet over medium-high heat until shimmering. Add the onion and ¼ teaspoon of the salt and cook for 5 to 7 minutes, or until softened and lightly browned. Transfer to a bowl.
3. Heat the remaining 1 tablespoon of the oil in now-empty skillet over medium-high heat until shimmering. Add the cabbage and sprinkle with

the remaining ½ teaspoon of the salt and black pepper. Cover and cook for about 3 minutes, without stirring, or until cabbage is wilted and lightly browned on bottom.
4. Stir and continue to cook for about 4 minutes, uncovered, or until the cabbage is crisp-tender and lightly browned in places, stirring once halfway through cooking. Off heat, stir in the cooked onion, parsley and lemon juice.
5. Transfer to a plate and serve.

Per Serving

calories: 117 | fat: 7.0g | protein: 2.7g | carbs: 13.4g | fiber: 5.1g | sodium: 472mg

Braised Cauliflower with White Wine

Prep time: 10 minutes | Cook time: 12 to 16 minutes | Serves 4 to 6

3 tablespoons plus 1 teaspoon extra-virgin olive oil, divided

3 garlic cloves, minced

1/8 teaspoon red pepper flakes

1 head cauliflower (2 pounds / 907 g), cored and cut into 1½-inch florets

¼ teaspoon salt, plus more for seasoning

Black pepper, to taste

1 cup vegetable broth

1/3 cup dry white wine

2 tablespoons minced fresh parsley

1. Combine 1 teaspoon of the oil, garlic and pepper flakes in small bowl.
2. Heat the remaining 3 tablespoons of the oil in a skillet over medium-high heat until shimmering. Add the cauliflower and ¼ teaspoon of the salt and cook for 7 to 9 minutes, stirring occasionally, or until florets are golden brown.
3. Push the cauliflower to sides of the skillet. Add the garlic mixture to the center of the skillet.

Cook for about 30 seconds, or until fragrant. Stir the garlic mixture into the cauliflower.
4. Pour in the broth and wine and bring to simmer. Reduce the heat to medium-low. Cover and cook for 4 to 6 minutes, or until the cauliflower is crisp-tender. Off heat, stir in the parsley and season with salt and pepper.
5. Serve immediately.

Per Serving

calories: 143 | fat: 11.7g | protein: 3.1g | carbs: 8.7g | fiber: 3.1g | sodium: 263mg

Cauliflower Steaks with Arugula

Prep time: 5 minutes | Cook time: 20 minutes | Serves 4

Cauliflower:

1 head cauliflower

Cooking spray

½ teaspoon garlic powder

4 cups arugula

Dressing:

1½ tablespoons extra-virgin olive oil

1½ tablespoons honey mustard

1 teaspoon freshly squeezed lemon juice

1. Preheat the oven to 425°F (220°C).
2. Remove the leaves from the cauliflower head, and cut it in half lengthwise. Cut 1½-inch-thick steaks from each half.
3. Spritz both sides of each steak with cooking spray and season both sides with the garlic powder.
4. Place the cauliflower steaks on a baking sheet, cover with foil, and roast in the oven for 10 minutes.
5. Remove the baking sheet from the oven and gently pull back the foil to avoid the steam. Flip the steaks, then roast uncovered for 10 minutes more.

6. Meanwhile, make the dressing: Whisk together the olive oil, honey mustard and lemon juice in a small bowl.
7. When the cauliflower steaks are done, divide into four equal portions. Top each portion with one-quarter of the arugula and dressing.
8. Serve immediately.

Per Serving

calories: 115 | fat: 6.0g | protein: 5.0g | carbs: 14.0g | fiber: 4.0g | sodium: 97mg

Parmesan Stuffed Zucchini Boats

Prep time: 5 minutes | Cook time: 15 minutes | Serves 4

1 cup canned low-sodium chickpeas, drained and rinsed

1 cup no-sugar-added spaghetti sauce

2 zucchinis

¼ cup shredded Parmesan cheese

1. Preheat the oven to 425ºF (220ºC).
2. In a medium bowl, stir together the chickpeas and spaghetti sauce.
3. Cut the zucchini in half lengthwise and scrape a spoon gently down the length of each half to remove the seeds.
4. Fill each zucchini half with the chickpea sauce and top with one-quarter of the Parmesan cheese.
5. Place the zucchini halves on a baking sheet and roast in the oven for 15 minutes.
6. Transfer to a plate. Let rest for 5 minutes before serving.

Per Serving

calories: 139 | fat: 4.0g | protein: 8.0g | carbs: 20.0g | fiber: 5.0g | sodium: 344mg

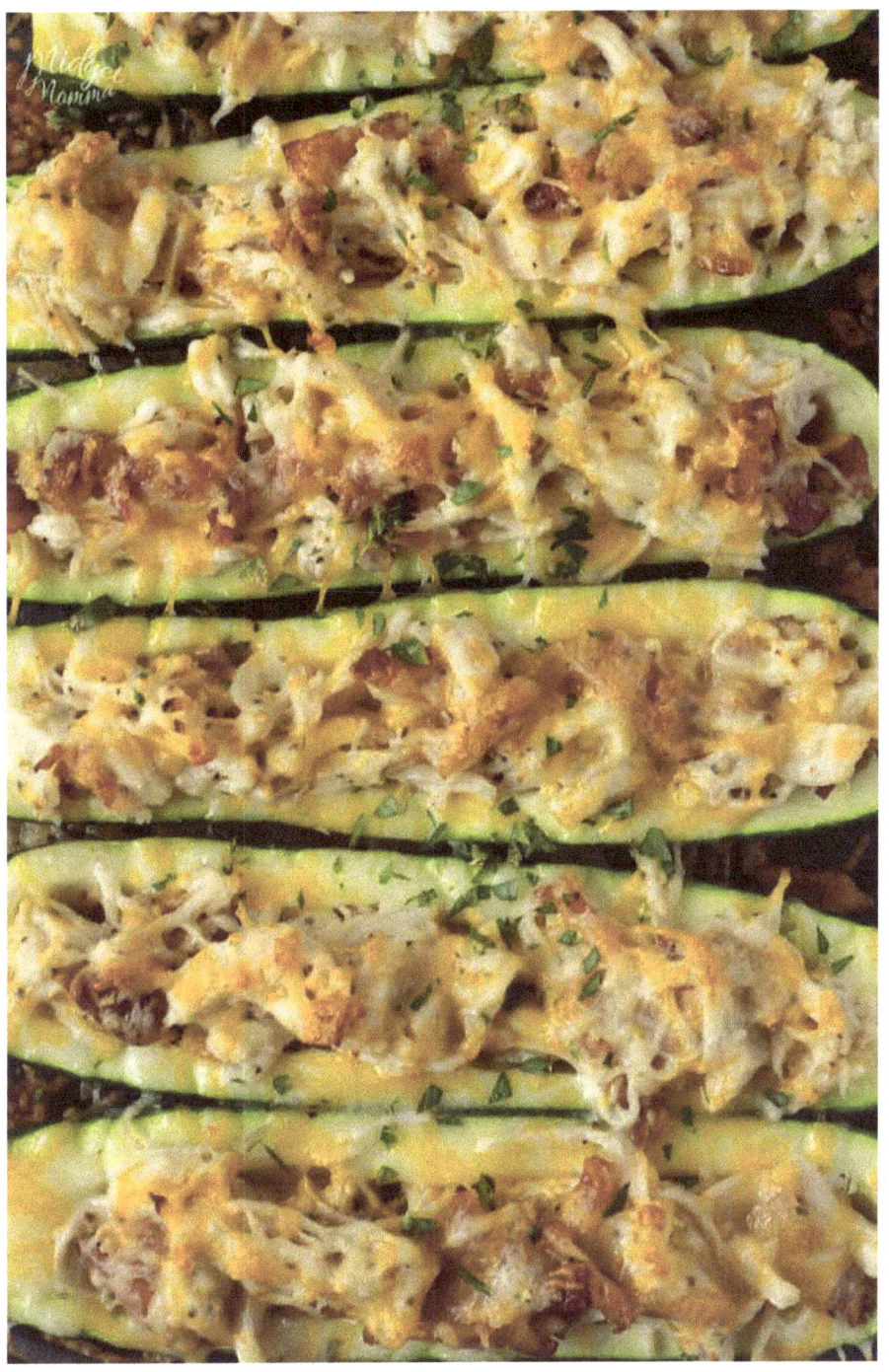

Baby Kale and Cabbage Salad

Prep time: 10 minutes | Cook time: 0 minutes | Serves 6

2 bunches baby kale, thinly sliced

½ head green savoy cabbage, cored and thinly sliced

1 medium red bell pepper, thinly sliced

1 garlic clove, thinly sliced

1 cup toasted peanuts

Dressing:

Juice of 1 lemon

¼ cup apple cider vinegar

1 teaspoon ground cumin

¼ teaspoon smoked paprika

1. In a large mixing bowl, toss together the kale and cabbage.
2. Make the dressing: Whisk together the lemon juice, vinegar, cumin and paprika in a small bowl.
3. Pour the dressing over the greens and gently massage with your hands.
4. Add the pepper, garlic and peanuts to the mixing bowl. Toss to combine.
5. Serve immediately.

Per Serving

calories: 199 | fat: 12.0g | protein: 10.0g | carbs: 17.0g | fiber: 5.0g | sodium: 46mg

Grilled Romaine Lettuce

Prep time: 5 minutes | Cook time: 3 to 5 minutes | Serves 4

Romaine:

2 heads romaine lettuce, halved lengthwise

2 tablespoons extra-virgin olive oil

Dressing:

½ cup unsweetened almond milk

1 tablespoon extra-virgin olive oil

¼ bunch fresh chives, thinly chopped

1 garlic clove, pressed

1 pinch red pepper flakes

1. Heat a grill pan over medium heat.
2. Brush each lettuce half with the olive oil. Place the lettuce halves, flat- side down, on the grill. Grill for 3 to 5 minutes, or until the lettuce slightly wilts and develops light grill marks.
3. Meanwhile, whisk together all the ingredients for the dressing in a small bowl.
4. Drizzle 2 tablespoons of the dressing over each romaine half and serve.

Per Serving

calories: 126 | fat: 11.0g | protein: 2.0g | carbs: 7.0g | fiber: 1.0g | sodium: 41mg

Mini Crustless Spinach Quiches

Prep time: 10 minutes | Cook time: 20 minutes | Serves 6

2 tablespoons extra-virgin olive oil

1 onion, finely chopped

2 cups baby spinach

2 garlic cloves, minced

8 large eggs, beaten

¼ cup unsweetened almond milk

½ teaspoon sea salt

¼ teaspoon freshly ground black pepper

1 cup shredded Swiss cheese

Cooking spray

1. Preheat the oven to 375ºF (190ºC). Spritz a 6-cup muffin tin with cooking spray. Set aside.
2. In a large skillet over medium-high heat, heat the olive oil until shimmering. Add the onion and cook for about 4 minutes, or until soft. Add the spinach and cook for about 1 minute, stirring constantly, or until the spinach softens. Add the garlic and sauté for 30 seconds. Remove from the heat and let cool.
3. In a medium bowl, whisk together the eggs, milk, salt and pepper.

4. Stir the cooled vegetables and the cheese into the egg mixture. Spoon the mixture into the prepared muffin tins. Bake for about 15 minutes, or until the eggs are set.
5. Let rest for 5 minutes before serving.

Per Serving

calories: 218 | fat: 17.0g | protein: 14.0g | carbs: 4.0g | fiber: 1.0g | sodium: 237mg

Butternut Noodles with Mushrooms

Prep time: 10 minutes | Cook time: 12 minutes | Serves 4

¼ cup extra-virgin olive oil

1 pound (454 g) cremini mushrooms, sliced

½ red onion, finely chopped

1 teaspoon dried thyme

½ teaspoon sea salt

3 garlic cloves, minced

½ cup dry white wine

Pinch of red pepper flakes

4 cups butternut noodles

4 ounces (113 g) grated Parmesan cheese

1. In a large skillet over medium-high heat, heat the olive oil until shimmering. Add the mushrooms, onion, thyme, and salt to the skillet. Cook for about 6 minutes, stirring occasionally, or until the mushrooms start to brown. Add the garlic and sauté for 30 seconds. Stir in the white wine and red pepper flakes.
2. Fold in the noodles. Cook for about 5 minutes, stirring occasionally, or until the noodles are tender.
3. Serve topped with the grated Parmesan.

Per Serving

calories: 244 | fat: 14.0g | protein: 4.0g | carbs: 22.0g | fiber: 4.0g | sodium: 159mg

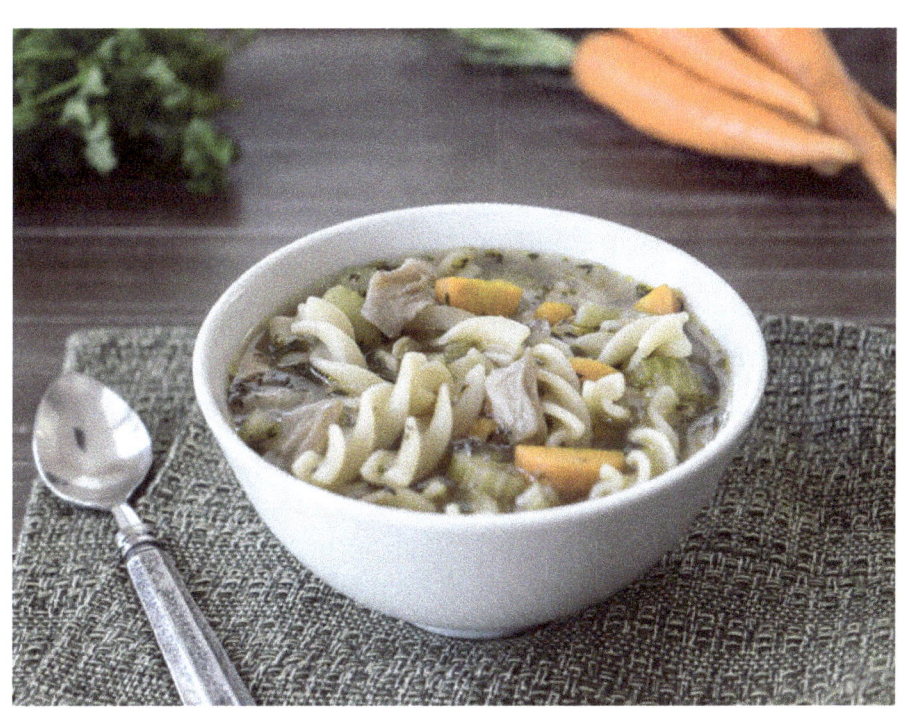

Potato Tortilla with Leeks and Mushrooms

Prep time: 30 minutes | Cook time: 50 minutes | Serves 2

1 tablespoon olive oil

1 cup thinly sliced leeks

4 ounces (113 g) baby bella (cremini) mushrooms, stemmed and sliced

1 small potato, peeled and sliced ¼-inch thick

½ cup unsweetened almond milk

5 large eggs, beaten

1 teaspoon Dijon mustard

½ teaspoon salt

½ teaspoon dried thyme

Pinch freshly ground black pepper

3 ounces (85 g) Gruyère cheese, shredded

1. Preheat the oven to 350ºF (180ºC).
2. In a large sauté pan over medium-high heat, heat the olive oil. Add the leeks, mushrooms, and potato and sauté for about 10 minutes, or until the potato starts to brown.

3. Reduce the heat to medium-low, cover, and cook for an additional 10 minutes, or until the potato begins to soften. Add 1 to 2 tablespoons of water to prevent sticking to the bottom of the pan, if needed.
4. Meanwhile, whisk together the milk, beaten eggs, mustard, salt, thyme, black pepper, and cheese in a medium bowl until combined.
5. When the potatoes are fork-tender, turn off the heat.
6. Transfer the cooked vegetables to an oiled nonstick ovenproof pan and arrange them in a nice layer along the bottom and slightly up the sides of the pan. Pour the milk mixture evenly over the vegetables.
7. Bake in the preheated oven for 25 to 30 minutes, or until the eggs are completely set and the top is golden and puffed.
8. Remove from the oven and cool for 5 minutes before cutting and serving.

Per Serving

calories: 541 | fat: 33.1g | protein: 32.8g | carbs: 31.0g | fiber: 4.0g | sodium: 912mg

Mushrooms Ragu with Cheesy Polenta

Prep time: 20 minutes | Cook time: 30 minutes | Serves 2

½ ounce (14 g) dried porcini mushrooms

1 pound (454 g) baby bella (cremini) mushrooms, quartered

2 tablespoons olive oil

1 garlic clove, minced

1 large shallot, minced

1 tablespoon flour

2 teaspoons tomato paste

½ cup red wine

1 cup mushroom stock (or reserved liquid from soaking the porcini mushrooms, if using)

1 fresh rosemary sprig

½ teaspoon dried thyme

1½ cups water

½ teaspoon salt, plus more as needed

1 cup instant polenta

2 tablespoons grated Parmesan cheese

1. Soak the dried porcini mushrooms in 1 cup of hot water for about 15 minutes to soften them. When ready, scoop them out of the water, reserving the soaking liquid. Mince the porcini mushrooms.

2. Heat the olive oil in a large sauté pan over medium-high heat. Add the mushrooms, garlic, and shallot and sauté for 10 minutes, or until the vegetables are beginning to caramelize.
3. Stir in the flour and tomato paste and cook for an additional 30 seconds. Add the red wine, mushroom stock, rosemary, and thyme. Bring the mixture to a boil, stirring constantly, or until it has thickened.
4. Reduce the heat and allow to simmer for 10 minutes.
5. Meanwhile, bring the water to a boil in a saucepan and sprinkle with the salt.
6. Add the instant polenta and stir quickly while it thickens. Scatter with the grated Parmesan cheese. Taste and season with more salt as needed. Serve warm.

Per Serving

calories: 450 | fat: 16.0g | protein: 14.1g | carbs: 57.8g | fiber: 5.0g | sodium: 165mg

Veggie Rice Bowls with Pesto Sauce

Prep time: 15 minutes | Cook time: 1 minute | Serves 2

- 2 cups water
- 1 cup arborio rice, rinsed
- Salt and ground black pepper, to taste
- 2 eggs
- 1 cup broccoli florets
- ½ pound (227 g) Brussels sprouts
- 1 carrot, peeled and chopped
- 1 small beet, peeled and cubed
- ¼ cup pesto sauce
- Lemon wedges, for serving

1. Combine the water, rice, salt, and pepper in the Instant Pot. Insert a trivet over rice and place a steamer basket on top. Add the eggs, broccoli, Brussels sprouts, carrots, beet cubes, salt, and pepper to the steamer basket.
2. Lock the lid. Select the Manual mode and set the cooking time for 1 minute at High Pressure.
3. When the timer beeps, perform a natural pressure release for 10 minutes, then release any remaining pressure. Carefully open the lid.

4. Remove the steamer basket and trivet from the pot and transfer the eggs to a bowl of ice water. Peel and halve the eggs. Use a fork to fluff the rice.
5. Divide the rice, broccoli, Brussels sprouts, carrot, beet cubes, and eggs into two bowls. Top with a dollop of pesto sauce and serve with the lemon wedges.

Per Serving

calories: 590 | fat: 34.1g | protein: 21.9g | carbs: 50.0g | fiber: 19.6g | sodium: 670mg

Roasted Cauliflower and Carrots

Prep time: 10 minutes | Cook time: 30 minutes | Serves 2

4 cups cauliflower florets (about ½ small head)

2 medium carrots, peeled, halved, and then sliced into quarters lengthwise

2 tablespoons olive oil, divided

½ teaspoon salt, divided

½ teaspoon garlic powder, divided

2 teaspoons za'atar spice mix, divided

1 (15-ounce / 425-g) can chickpeas, drained, rinsed, and patted dry

¾ cup plain Greek yogurt

1 teaspoon harissa spice paste, plus additional as needed

1. Preheat the oven to 400ºF (205ºC). Line a sheet pan with foil or parchment paper.
2. Put the cauliflower and carrots in a large bowl. Drizzle with 1 tablespoon of olive oil and sprinkle with ¼ teaspoon of salt, ¼ teaspoon of garlic powder, and 1 teaspoon of za'atar. Toss to combine well.
3. Spread the vegetables onto one half of the prepared sheet pan in a single layer.

4. Put the chickpeas in the same bowl and season with the remaining 1 tablespoon of olive oil, ¼ teaspoon of salt, ¼ teaspoon of garlic powder, and the remaining 1 teaspoon of za'atar. Toss to combine well.
5. Spread the chickpeas onto the other half of the sheet pan.
6. Roast in the preheated oven for 30 minutes, or until the vegetables are crisp-tender. Flip the vegetables halfway through and give the chickpeas a stir so they cook evenly.
7. Meanwhile, whisk the yogurt and harissa together in a small bowl. Taste and add additional harissa as needed.
8. Serve the vegetables and chickpeas with the yogurt mixture on the side.

Per Serving

calories: 468 | fat: 23.0g | protein: 18.1g | carbs: 54.1g | fiber: 13.8g | sodium: 631mg

Sauté ed Spinach and Leeks

Prep time: 5 minutes | Cook time: 8 minutes | Serves 2

- 3 tablespoons olive oil
- 2 garlic cloves, crushed
- 2 leeks, chopped
- 2 red onions, chopped
- 9 ounces (255 g) fresh spinach
- 1 teaspoon kosher salt
- ½ cup crumbled goat cheese

1. Coat the bottom of the Instant Pot with the olive oil.
2. Add the garlic, leek, and onions and stir-fry for about 5 minutes, on Sauté mode.
3. Stir in the spinach. Sprinkle with the salt and sauté for an additional 3 minutes, stirring constantly.
4. Transfer to a plate and scatter with the goat cheese before serving.

Per Serving

calories: 447 | fat: 31.2g | protein: 14.6g | carbs: 28.7g | fiber: 6.3g | sodium: 937mg

Zoodles with Beet Pesto

Prep time: 10 minutes | Cook time: 50 minutes | Serves 2

1 medium red beet, peeled, chopped

½ cup walnut pieces

½ cup crumbled goat cheese

3 garlic cloves

2 tablespoons freshly squeezed lemon juice

2 tablespoons plus 2 teaspoons extra-virgin olive oil, divided

¼ teaspoon salt

4 small zucchinis, spiralized

1. Preheat the oven to 375ºF (190ºC).
2. Wrap the chopped beet in a piece of aluminum foil and seal well.
3. Roast in the preheated oven for 30 to 40 minutes until tender.
4. Meanwhile, heat a skillet over medium-high heat until hot. Add the walnuts and toast for 5 to 7 minutes, or until fragrant and lightly browned.
5. Remove the cooked beets from the oven and place in a food processor. Add the toasted walnuts, goat cheese, garlic, lemon juice, 2

tablespoons of olive oil, and salt. Pulse until smoothly blended. Set aside.
6. Heat the remaining 2 teaspoons of olive oil in a large skillet over medium heat. Add the zucchini and toss to coat in the oil. Cook for 2 to 3 minutes, stirring gently, or until the zucchini is softened.
7. Transfer the zucchini to a serving plate and toss with the beet pesto, then serve.

Per Serving

calories: 423 | fat: 38.8g | protein: 8.0g | carbs: 17.1g | fiber: 6.0g | sodium: 338mg

Fried Eggplant Rolls

Prep time: 20 minutes | Cook time: 10 minutes | Serves 4 to 6

1 large eggplants, trimmed and cut lengthwise into ¼-inch-thick slices

1 teaspoon salt

1 cup ricotta cheese

4 ounces (113 g) goat cheese, shredded

¼ cup finely chopped fresh basil

½ teaspoon freshly ground black pepper

Olive oil spray

1. Add the eggplant slices to a colander and season with salt. Set aside for 15 to 20 minutes.
2. Mix together the ricotta and goat cheese, basil, and black pepper in a large bowl and stir to combine. Set aside.
3. Dry the eggplant slices with paper towels and lightly mist them with olive oil spray.
4. Heat a large skillet over medium heat and lightly spray it with olive oil spray.
5. Arrange the eggplant slices in the skillet and fry each side for 3 minutes until golden brown.

6. Remove from the heat to a paper towel-lined plate and rest for 5 minutes.
7. Make the eggplant rolls: Lay the eggplant slices on a flat work surface and top each slice with a tablespoon of the prepared cheese mixture. Roll them up and serve immediately.

Per Serving

calories: 254 | fat: 14.9g | protein: 15.3g | carbs: 18.6g | fiber: 7.1g | sodium: 745mg

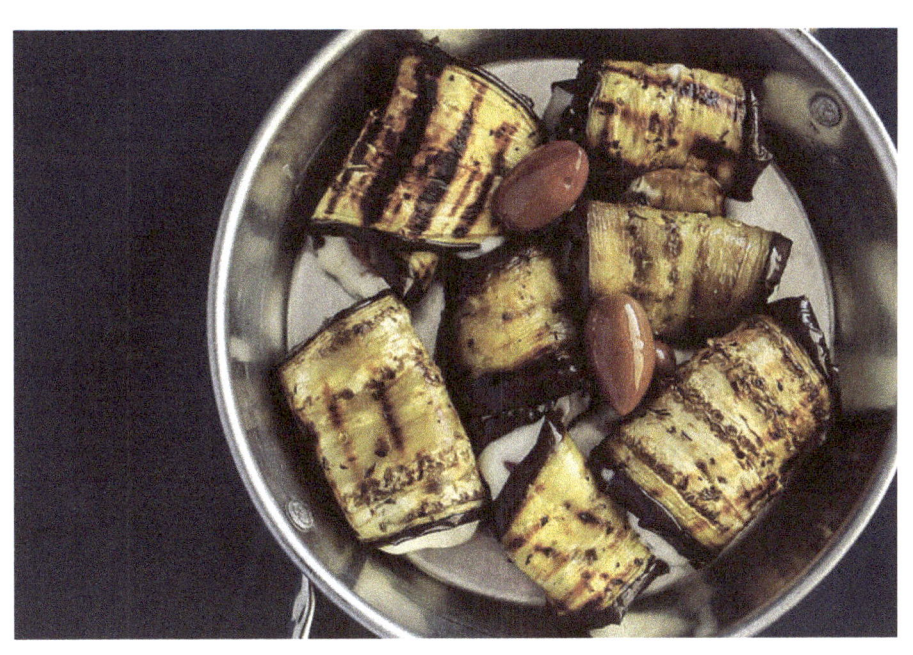

Garlicky Zucchini Cubes with Mint

Prep time: 5 minutes | Cook time: 10 minutes | Serves 4

- 3 large green zucchini, cut into ½-inch cubes
- 3 tablespoons extra-virgin olive oil
- 1 large onion, chopped
- 3 cloves garlic, minced
- 1 teaspoon salt
- 1 teaspoon dried mint

1. Heat the olive oil in a large skillet over medium heat.
2. Add the onion and garlic and sauté for 3 minutes, stirring constantly, or until softened.
3. Stir in the zucchini cubes and salt and cook for 5 minutes, or until the zucchini is browned and tender.
4. Add the mint to the skillet and toss to combine, then continue cooking for 2 minutes.
5. Serve warm.

Per Serving

calories: 146 | fat: 10.6g | protein: 4.2g | carbs: 11.8g | fiber: 3.0g | sodium: 606mg

Zucchini and Artichokes Bowl with Farro

Prep time: 15 minutes | Cook time: 10 minutes | Serves 4 to 6

1/3 cup extra-virgin olive oil

1/3 cup chopped red onions

1/2 cup chopped red bell pepper

2 garlic cloves, minced

1 cup zucchini, cut into 1/2-inch-thick slices

1/2 cup coarsely chopped artichokes

1/2 cup canned chickpeas, drained and rinsed

3 cups cooked farro

Salt and freshly ground black pepper, to taste

1/2 cup crumbled feta cheese, for serving (optional)

1/4 cup sliced olives, for serving (optional)

2 tablespoons fresh basil, chiffonade, for serving (optional)

3 tablespoons balsamic vinegar, for serving (optional)

1. Heat the olive oil in a large skillet over medium heat until it shimmers.

2. Add the onions, bell pepper, and garlic and sauté for 5 minutes, stirring occasionally, until softened.
3. Stir in the zucchini slices, artichokes, and chickpeas and sauté for about 5 minutes until slightly tender.
4. Add the cooked farro and toss to combine until heated through. Sprinkle the salt and pepper to season.
5. Divide the mixture into bowls. Top each bowl evenly with feta cheese, olive slices, and basil and sprinkle with the balsamic vinegar, if desired.

Per Serving

calories: 366 | fat: 19.9g | protein: 9.3g | carbs: 50.7g | fiber: 9.0g | sodium: 86mg

Zucchini Fritters

Prep time: 15 minutes | Cook time: 5 minutes | Makes 14 fritters

- 4 cups grated zucchini
- Salt, to taste
- 2 large eggs, lightly beaten
- 1/3 cup sliced scallions (green and white parts)
- 2/3 all-purpose flour
- 1/8 teaspoon black pepper
- 2 tablespoons olive oil

1. Put the grated zucchini in a colander and lightly season with salt. Set aside to rest for 10 minutes. Squeeze out as much liquid from the grated zucchini as possible.
2. Pour the grated zucchini into a bowl. Fold in the beaten eggs, scallions, flour, salt, and pepper and stir until everything is well combined.
3. Heat the olive oil in a large skillet over medium heat until hot.
4. Drop 3 tablespoons mounds of the zucchini mixture onto the hot skillet to make each fritter, pressing them lightly into rounds and spacing them about 2 inches apart.

5. Cook for 2 to 3 minutes. Flip the zucchini fritters and cook for 2 minutes more, or until they are golden brown and cooked through.
6. Remove from the heat to a plate lined with paper towels. Repeat with the remaining zucchini mixture.
7. Serve hot.

Per Serving (2 fritters)

calories: 113 | fat: 6.1g | protein: 4.0g | carbs: 12.2g | fiber: 1.0g | sodium: 25mg

Fish and Seafood

Mussels with Onions

Prep time: 10 minutes | Cook time: 7 minutes | Serves 8

2 tablespoons olive oil

2 medium yellow onions, chopped

1 teaspoon dried rosemary, crushed

2 garlic cloves, minced

2 cups chicken broth

4 pounds (1.8 kg) mussels, cleaned and debearded

¼ cup fresh lemon juice

Salt and ground black pepper as needed

1. Put the oil to the Instant Pot and select the Sauté function for cooking.
2. Add the onions and cook for 5 minutes with occasional stirring.
3. Add the rosemary and garlic to the pot. Stir and cook for 1 minute.
4. Pour the chicken broth and lemon juice into the cooker, sprinkle some salt and black pepper over it.
5. Place the trivet inside the cooker and arrange the mussels over it.

6. Select the Manual function at Low Pressure for 1 minute.
7. Secure the lid and let the mussels cook.
8. After the beep, do a Quick release then remove the lid.
9. Serve the mussels with its steaming hot soup in a bowl.

Per Serving

calories: 249 | fat: 8.8g | protein: 28.5g | carbs: 11.9g | fiber: 0.5g | sodium: 844mg

Cod Curry

Prep time: 5 minutes | Cook time: 12 minutes | Serves 8

- 3 pounds (1.4 kg) cod fillets, cut into bite-sized pieces
- 2 tablespoons olive oil
- 4 curry leaves
- 4 medium onions, chopped
- 2 tablespoons fresh ginger, grated finely
- 4 garlic cloves, minced
- 4 tablespoons curry powder
- 4 teaspoons ground cumin
- 4 teaspoons ground coriander
- 2 teaspoons red chili powder
- 1 teaspoon ground turmeric
- 4 cups unsweetened coconut milk
- 2½ cups tomatoes, chopped
- 2 Serrano peppers, seeded and chopped
- 2 tablespoons fresh lemon juice

1. Add the oil to the Instant Pot and select Sauté function for cooking.
2. Add the curry leaves and cook for 30 seconds. Stir the onion, garlic, and ginger into the pot and cook 5 minutes.

3. Add all the spices to the mixture and cook for another 1½ minutes.
4. Hit Cancel then add the coconut milk, Serrano pepper, tomatoes, and fish to the pot.
5. Secure the lid and select the Manual settings with Low Pressure and 5 minutes cooking time.
6. After the beep, do a Quick release and remove the lid.
7. Drizzle lemon juice over the curry then stir.
8. Serve immediately.

Per Serving

calories: 424 | fat: 29.1g | protein: 30.2g | carbs: 14.4g | fiber: 3.8g | sodium: 559mg

Shrimps with Northern Beans

Prep time: 10 minutes | Cook time: 25 minutes | Serves 3

1½ tablespoons olive oil
1 medium onion, chopped
½ small green bell pepper, seeded and chopped
½ celery stalk, chopped
1 garlic clove, minced
1 tablespoon fresh parsley, chopped
½ teaspoon red pepper flakes, crushed
½ teaspoon cayenne pepper
½ pound (227 g) great northern beans, rinsed, soaked, and drained
1 cup chicken broth
1 bay leaf
½ pound (227 g) medium shrimp, peeled and deveined

1. Select the Sauté function on your Instant pot, then add the oil, onion, celery, bell pepper and cook for 5 minutes.
2. Now add the parsley, garlic, spices, and bay leaf to the pot and cook for another 2 minutes.
3. Pour in the chicken broth then add the beans to it. Secure the cooker lid.

4. Select the Manual function for 15 minutes with medium pressure.
5. After the beep, do a Natural release for 10 minutes and remove the lid.
6. Add the shrimp to the beans and cook them together on the Manual function for 2 minutes at High Pressure.
7. Do a Quick release, keep it aside for 10 minutes, then remove the lid.
8. Serve hot.

Per Serving

calories: 405 | fat: 9.1g | protein: 29.1g | carbs: 53.1g | fiber: 16.4g | sodium: 702mg

Shrimp and Potato Curry

Prep time: 5 minutes | Cook time: 9 minutes | Serves 8

- 2 tablespoons olive oil
- 1½ medium onions, chopped
- 1½ teaspoons ground cumin
- 2 teaspoons red chili powder
- 2 teaspoons ground turmeric
- 3 medium white rose potatoes, diced
- 6 medium tomatoes, chopped
- 2 pounds (907 g) medium shrimp, peeled and deveined
- 1½ tablespoons fresh lemon juice
- Salt, to taste
- ½ cup fresh cilantro, chopped

1. Select the Sauté function on your Instant Pot. Add the oil and onions then cook for 2 minutes.
2. Add the tomatoes, potatoes, cilantro, lemon juice and all the spices into the pot and secure the lid.
3. Select the Manual function at medium pressure for 5 minutes.
4. Do a natural release then remove the lid. Stir shrimp into the pot.

5. Secure the lid again then set the Manual function with High Pressure for 2 minutes.
6. After the beep, use Natural release and let it stand for 10 minutes.
7. Remove the lid and serve hot.

Per Serving

calories: 197 | fat: 5.0g | protein: 18.1g | carbs: 20.3g | fiber: 3.9g | sodium: 700mg

Sardines and Plum Tomato Curry

Prep time: 10 minutes | Cook time: 8 hours 2 minutes | Serves 4

1 tablespoon olive oil
1 pound (454 g) fresh sardines, cubed
2 plum tomatoes, chopped finely
½ large onion, sliced
1 garlic clove, minced
½ cup tomato purée
Salt and ground black pepper, to taste

1. Select the Sauté function on your Instant pot then add the oil and sardines to it.
2. Let it sauté for 2 minutes then add all the remaining ingredients.
3. Cover the lid and select Slow Cook function for 8 hours.
4. Remove the lid and stir the cooked curry.
5. Serve warm.

Per Serving

calories: 292 | fat: 16.5g | protein: 28.9g | carbs: 6.0g | fiber: 1.3g | sodium: 398mg

Salmon and Mushroom Hash with Pesto

Prep time: 15 minutes | Cook time: 20 minutes | Serves 6

Pesto:

¼ cup extra-virgin olive oil

1 bunch fresh basil

Juice and zest of 1 lemon

1 cup water

¼ teaspoon salt, plus additional as needed

Hash:

2 tablespoons extra-virgin olive oil

6 cups mixed mushrooms (brown, white, shiitake, cremini, portobello, etc.), sliced

1 pound (454 g) wild salmon, cubed

1. Make the pesto: Pulse the olive oil, basil, juice and zest, water, and salt in a blender or food processor until smoothly blended. Set aside.
2. Heat the olive oil in a large skillet over medium heat.
3. Stir-fry the mushrooms for 6 to 8 minutes, or until they begin to exude their juices.

4. Add the salmon and cook each side for 5 to 6 minutes until cooked through.
5. Fold in the prepared pesto and stir well. Taste and add additional salt as needed. Serve warm.

Per Serving

calories: 264 | fat: 14.7g | protein: 7.0g | carbs: 30.9g | fiber: 4.0g | sodium: 480mg

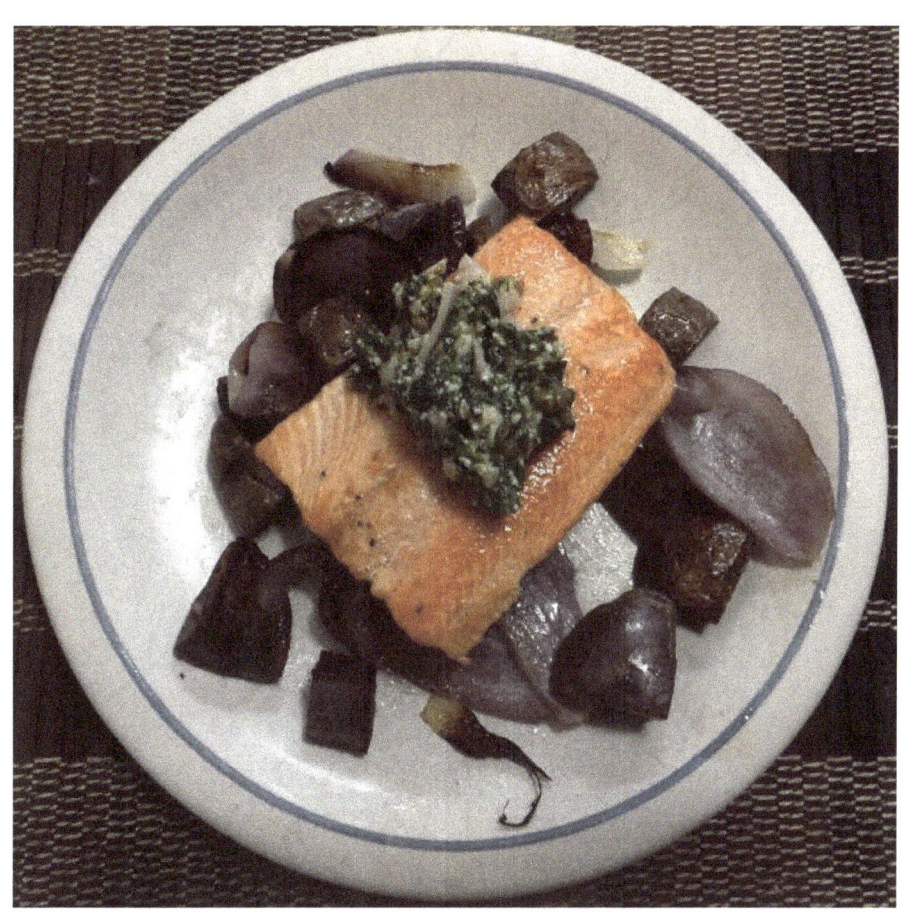

Spiced Citrus Sole

Prep time: 10 minutes | Cook time: 10 minutes | Serves 4

- 1 teaspoon garlic powder
- 1 teaspoon chili powder
- ½ teaspoon lemon zest
- ½ teaspoon lime zest
- ¼ teaspoon smoked paprika
- ¼ teaspoon freshly ground black pepper Pinch sea salt
- 4 (6-ounce / 170-g) sole fillets, patted dry
- 1 tablespoon extra-virgin olive oil
- 2 teaspoons freshly squeezed lime juice

1. Preheat the oven to 450°F (235°C). Line a baking sheet with aluminum foil and set aside.
2. Mix together the garlic powder, chili powder, lemon zest, lime zest, paprika, pepper, and salt in a small bowl until well combined.
3. Arrange the sole fillets on the prepared baking sheet and rub the spice mixture all over the fillets until well coated. Drizzle the olive oil and lime juice over the fillets.

4. Bake in the preheated oven for about 8 minutes until flaky.
5. Remove from the heat to a plate and serve.

Per Serving

calories: 183 | fat: 5.0g | protein: 32.1g | carbs: 0g | fiber: 0g | sodium: 136mg

Asian-Inspired Tuna Lettuce Wraps

Prep time: 10 minutes | Cook time: 0 minutes | Serves 2

¼ cup almond butter
1 tablespoon freshly squeezed lemon juice
1 teaspoon low-sodium soy sauce
1 teaspoon curry powder
½ teaspoon sriracha, or to taste
½ cup canned water chestnuts, drained and chopped
2 (2.6-ounce / 74-g) package tuna packed in water, drained
2 large butter lettuce leaves

1. Stir together the almond butter, lemon juice, soy sauce, curry powder, sriracha in a medium bowl until well mixed. Add the water chestnuts and tuna and stir until well incorporated.
2. Place 2 butter lettuce leaves on a flat work surface, spoon half of the tuna mixture onto each leaf and roll up into a wrap. Serve immediately.

Per Serving

calories: 270 | fat: 13.9g | protein: 19.1g | carbs: 18.5g | fiber: 3.0g | sodium: 626mg

Crispy Tilapia with Mango Salsa

Prep time: 5 minutes | Cook time: 10 minutes | Serves 2

Salsa:
1 cup chopped mango
2 tablespoons chopped fresh cilantro
2 tablespoons chopped red onion
2 tablespoons freshly squeezed lime juice
½ jalapeño pepper, seeded and minced
Pinch salt

Tilapia:
1 tablespoon paprika
1 teaspoon onion powder
½ teaspoon dried thyme
½ teaspoon freshly ground black pepper
¼ teaspoon cayenne pepper
½ teaspoon garlic powder
¼ teaspoon salt
½ pound (227 g) boneless tilapia fillets
2 teaspoons extra-virgin olive oil
1 lime, cut into wedges, for serving

1. Make the salsa: Place the mango, cilantro, onion, lime juice, jalapeño, and salt in a medium bowl and toss to combine. Set aside.
2. Make the tilapia: Stir together the paprika, onion powder, thyme, black pepper, cayenne

pepper, garlic powder, and salt in a small bowl until well mixed. Rub both sides of fillets generously with the mixture.
3. Heat the olive oil in a large skillet over medium heat.
4. Add the fish fillets and cook each side for 3 to 5 minutes until golden brown and cooked through.
5. Divide the fillets among two plates and spoon half of the prepared salsa onto each fillet. Serve the fish alongside the lime wedges.

Per Serving

calories: 239 | fat: 7.8g | protein: 25.0g | carbs: 21.9g | fiber: 4.0g | sodium: 416mg

Mediterranean Grilled Sea Bass

Prep time: 20 minutes | Cook time: 20 minutes | Serves 6

¼ teaspoon onion powder
¼ teaspoon garlic powder
¼ teaspoon paprika
Lemon pepper and sea salt to taste
2 pounds (907 g) sea bass
3 tablespoons extra-virgin olive oil, divided
2 large cloves garlic, chopped
1 tablespoon chopped Italian flat leaf parsley

1. Preheat the grill to high heat.
2. Place the onion powder, garlic powder, paprika, lemon pepper, and sea salt in a large bowl and stir to combine.
3. Dredge the fish in the spice mixture, turning until well coated.
4. Heat 2 tablespoon of olive oil in a small skillet. Add the garlic and parsley and cook for 1 to 2 minutes, stirring occasionally. Remove the skillet from the heat and set aside.
5. Brush the grill grates lightly with remaining 1 tablespoon olive oil.

6. Grill the fish for about 7 minutes. Flip the fish and drizzle with the garlic mixture and cook for an additional 7 minutes, or until the fish flakes when pressed lightly with a fork.
7. Serve hot.

Per Serving

calories: 200 | fat: 10.3g | protein: 26.9g | carbs: 0.6g | fiber: 0.1g | sodium: 105mg

Braised Branzino with Wine Sauce

Prep time: 15 minutes | Cook time: 15 minutes | Serves 2 to 3

Sauce:

¾ cup dry white wine

2 tablespoons white wine vinegar

2 tablespoons cornstarch

1 tablespoon honey

Fish:

1 large branzino, butterflied and patted dry

2 tablespoons onion powder

2 tablespoons paprika

½ tablespoon salt

6 tablespoons extra-virgin olive oil, divided

4 garlic cloves, thinly sliced

4 scallions, both green and white parts, thinly sliced

1 large tomato, cut into ¼-inch cubes

4 kalamata olives, pitted and chopped

1. Make the sauce: Mix together the white wine, vinegar, cornstarch, and honey in a bowl and keep stirring until the honey has dissolved. Set aside.
2. Make the fish: Place the fish on a clean work surface, skin-side down. Sprinkle the onion

powder, paprika, and salt to season. Drizzle 2 tablespoons of olive oil all over the fish.
3. Heat 2 tablespoons of olive oil in a large skillet over high heat until it shimmers.
4. Add the fish, skin-side up, to the skillet and brown for about 2 minutes. Carefully flip the fish and cook for another 3 minutes. Remove from the heat to a plate and set aside.
5. Add the remaining 2 tablespoons olive oil to the skillet and swirl to coat. Stir in the garlic cloves, scallions, tomato, and kalamata olives and sauté for 5 minutes. Pour in the prepared sauce and stir to combine.
6. Return the fish (skin-side down) to the skillet, flipping to coat in the sauce. Reduce the heat to medium-low, and cook for an additional 5 minutes until cooked through.
7. Using a slotted spoon, transfer the fish to a plate and serve warm.

Per Serving

calories: 1059 | fat: 71.9g | protein: 46.2g | carbs: 55.8g | fiber: 5.1g | sodium: 2807mg

Peppercorn-Seared Tuna Steaks

Prep time: 5 minutes | Cook time: 10 minutes | Serves 2

2 (5-ounce / 142-g) ahi tuna steaks

1 teaspoon kosher salt

¼ teaspoon cayenne pepper

2 tablespoons olive oil

1 teaspoon whole peppercorns

1. On a plate, Season the tuna steaks on both sides with salt and cayenne pepper.
2. In a skillet, heat the olive oil over medium-high heat until it shimmers.
3. Add the peppercorns and cook for about 5 minutes, or until they soften and pop.
4. Carefully put the tuna steaks in the skillet and sear for 1 to 2 minutes per side, depending on the thickness of the tuna steaks, or until the fish is cooked to the desired level of doneness.
5. Cool for 5 minutes before serving.

Per Serving

calories: 260 | fat: 14.3g | protein: 33.4g | carbs: 0.2g | fiber: 0.1g | sodium: 1033mg

Canned Sardine Donburi (Rice Bowl)

Prep time: 10 minutes | Cook time: 40 to 50 minutes | Serves 4 to 6

- 4 cups water
- 2 cups brown rice, rinsed well
- ½ teaspoon salt
- 3 (4-ounce / 113-g) cans sardines packed in water, drained
- 3 scallions, sliced thin
- 1-inch piece fresh ginger, grated
- 4 tablespoons sesame oil

1. Place the water, brown rice, and salt to a large saucepan and stir to combine. Allow the mixture to boil over high heat.
2. Once boiling, reduce the heat to low, and cook covered for 45 to 50 minutes, or until the rice is tender.
3. Meanwhile, roughly mash the sardines with a fork in a medium bowl.
4. When the rice is done, stir in the mashed sardines, scallions, and ginger.
5. Divide the mixture into four bowls. Top each bowl with a drizzle of sesame oil. Serve warm.

Per Serving

calories: 603 | fat: 23.6g | protein: 25.2g | carbs: 73.8g | fiber: 4.0g | sodium: 498mg

Baked Halibut Steaks with Vegetables

Prep time: 15 minutes | Cook time: 20 minutes | Serves 4

2 teaspoon olive oil, divided

1 clove garlic, peeled and minced

½ cup minced onion

1 cup diced zucchini

2 cups diced fresh tomatoes

2 tablespoons chopped fresh basil

¼ teaspoon salt

¼ teaspoon ground black pepper

4 (6-ounce / 170-g) halibut steaks

1 cup crumbled feta cheese

1. Preheat oven to 450ºF (235ºC). Coat a shallow baking dish lightly with 1 teaspoon of olive oil.
2. In a medium saucepan, heat the remaining 1 teaspoon of olive oil.
3. Add the garlic, onion, and zucchini and mix well. Cook for 5 minutes, stirring occasionally, or until the zucchini is softened.
4. Remove the saucepan from the heat and stir in the tomatoes, basil, salt, and pepper.

5. Place the halibut steaks in the coated baking dish in a single layer. Spread the zucchini mixture evenly over the steaks. Scatter the top with feta cheese.
6. Bake in the preheated oven for about 15 minutes, or until the fish flakes when pressed lightly with a fork. Serve hot.

Per Serving

calories: 258 | fat: 7.6g | protein: 38.6g | carbs: 6.5g | fiber: 1.2g | sodium: 384mg Fish and Seafood

Spicy Haddock Stew

Prep time: 15 minutes | Cook time: 35 minutes | Serves 6

- ¼ cup coconut oil
- 1 tablespoon minced garlic
- 1 onion, chopped
- 2 celery stalks, chopped
- ½ fennel bulb, thinly sliced
- 1 carrot, diced
- 1 sweet potato, diced
- 1 (15-ounce / 425-g) can low-sodium diced tomatoes
- 1 cup coconut milk
- 1 cup low-sodium chicken broth
- ¼ teaspoon red pepper flakes
- 12 ounces (340 g) haddock, cut into 1-inch chunks
- 2 tablespoons chopped fresh cilantro, for garnish

1. In a large saucepan, heat the coconut oil over medium-high heat.
2. Add the garlic, onion, and celery and sauté for about 4 minutes, stirring occasionally, or until they are tender.
3. Stir in the fennel bulb, carrot, and sweet potato and sauté for 4 minutes more.

4. Add the diced tomatoes, coconut milk, chicken broth, and red pepper flakes and stir to incorporate, then bring the mixture to a boil.
5. Once it starts to boil, reduce the heat to low, and bring to a simmer for about 15 minutes, or until the vegetables are fork-tender.
6. Add the haddock chunks and continue simmering for about 10 minutes, or until the fish is cooked through.
7. Sprinkle the cilantro on top for garnish before serving.

Per Serving

calories: 276 | fat: 20.9g | protein: 14.2g | carbs: 6.8g | fiber: 3.0g | sodium: 226mg

Orange Flavored Scallops

Prep time: 10 minutes | Cook time: 10 minutes | Serves 4

- 2 pounds (907 g) sea scallops, patted dry
- Sea salt and freshly ground black pepper, to taste
- 2 tablespoons extra-virgin olive oil
- 1 tablespoon minced garlic
- ¼ cup freshly squeezed orange juice
- 1 teaspoon orange zest
- 2 teaspoons chopped fresh thyme, for garnish

1. In a bowl, lightly season the scallops with salt and pepper. Set aside.
2. Heat the olive oil in a large skillet over medium-high heat until it shimmers.
3. Add the garlic and sauté for about 3 minutes, or until fragrant.
4. Stir in the seasoned scallops and sear each side for about 4 minutes, or until the scallops are browned.
5. Remove the scallops from the heat to a plate and set aside.
6. Add the orange juice and zest to the skillet, scraping up brown bits from bottom of skillet.

7. Drizzle the sauce over the scallops and garnish with the thyme before serving.

Per Serving

calories: 266 | fat: 7.6g | protein: 38.1g | carbs: 7.9g | fiber: 0g | sodium: 360mg

Garlic Skillet Salmon

Prep time: 5 minutes | Cook time: 14 to 16 minutes | Serves 4

1 tablespoon extra-virgin olive oil
2 garlic cloves, minced
1 teaspoon smoked paprika
1½ cups grape or cherry tomatoes, quartered
1 (12-ounce / 340-g) jar roasted red peppers, drained and chopped
1 tablespoon water
¼ teaspoon freshly ground black pepper
¼ teaspoon kosher or sea salt
1 pound (454 g) salmon fillets, skin removed and cut into 8 pieces
1 tablespoon freshly squeezed lemon juice

1. In a large skillet over medium heat, heat the oil. Add the garlic and smoked paprika and cook for 1 minute, stirring often. Add the tomatoes, roasted peppers, water, black pepper, and salt. Turn up the heat to medium-high, bring to a simmer, and cook for 3 minutes, stirring occasionally and smashing the tomatoes with a wooden spoon toward the end of the cooking time.
2. Add the salmon to the skillet, and spoon some of the sauce over the top. Cover and cook for

10 to 12 minutes, or until the salmon is cooked through and just starts to flake.
3. Remove the skillet from the heat, and drizzle lemon juice over the top of the fish. Stir the sauce, then break up the salmon into chunks with a fork. Serve hot.

Per Serving

calories: 255 | fat: 11.7g | protein: 24.2g | carbs: 5.9g | fiber: 1.2g | sodium: 809mg

Fruits and Desserts

Chocolate, Almond, and Cherry Clusters

Prep time: 15 minutes | Cook time: 3 minutes | Makes 10 clusters

1 cup dark chocolate (60% cocoa or higher), chopped

1 tablespoon coconut oil

½ cup dried cherries

1 cup roasted salted almonds

1. Line a baking sheet with parchment paper.
2. Melt the chocolate and coconut oil in a saucepan for 3 minutes. Stir constantly.
3. Turn off the heat and mix in the cherries and almonds.
4. Drop the mixture on the baking sheet with a spoon. Place the sheet in the refrigerator and chill for at least 1 hour or until firm.
5. Serve chilled.

Per Serving

calories: 197 | fat: 13.2g | protein: 4.1g | carbs: 17.8g | fiber: 4.0g | sodium: 57mg

Chocolate and Avocado Mousse

Prep time: 40 minutes | Cook time: 5 minutes | Serves 4 to 6

8 ounces (227 g) dark chocolate (60% cocoa or higher), chopped

¼ cup unsweetened coconut milk

2 tablespoons coconut oil

2 ripe avocados, deseeded

¼ cup raw honey

Sea salt, to taste

1. Put the chocolate in a saucepan. Pour in the coconut milk and add the coconut oil.
2. Cook for 3 minutes or until the chocolate and coconut oil melt. Stir constantly.
3. Put the avocado in a food processor, then drizzle with honey and melted chocolate. Pulse to combine until smooth.
4. Pour the mixture in a serving bowl, then sprinkle with salt. Refrigerate to chill for 30 minutes and serve.

Per Serving

calories: 654 | fat: 46.8g | protein: 7.2g | carbs: 55.9g | fiber: 9.0g | sodium: 112mg

Coconut Blueberries with Brown Rice

Prep time: 55 minutes | Cook time: 10 minutes | Serves 4

1 cup fresh blueberries	¼ cup maple syrup
2 cups unsweetened coconut milk	Sea salt, to taste
1 teaspoon ground ginger	2 cups cooked brown rice

1. Put all the ingredients, except for the brown rice, in a pot. Stir to combine well.
2. Cook over medium-high heat for 7 minutes or until the blueberries are tender.
3. Pour in the brown rice and cook for 3 more minute or until the rice is soft. Stir constantly.
4. Serve immediately.

Per Serving

calories: 470 | fat: 24.8g | protein: 6.2g | carbs: 60.1g | fiber: 5.0g | sodium: 75mg

Blueberry and Oat Crisp

Prep time: 15 minutes | Cook time: 20 minutes | Serves 4

- 2 tablespoons coconut oil, melted, plus more for greasing
- 4 cups fresh blueberries
- Juice of ½ lemon
- 2 teaspoons lemon zest
- ¼ cup maple syrup
- 1 cup gluten-free rolled oats
- ½ cup chopped pecans
- ½ teaspoon ground cinnamon
- Sea salt, to taste

1. Preheat the oven to 350°F (180°C). Grease a baking sheet with coconut oil.
2. Combine the blueberries, lemon juice and zest, and maple syrup in a bowl. Stir to mix well, then spread the mixture on the baking sheet.
3. Combine the remaining ingredients in a small bowl. Stir to mix well. Pour the mixture over the blueberries mixture.
4. Bake in the preheated oven for 20 minutes or until the oats are golden brown.
5. Serve immediately with spoons.

Per Serving

calories: 496 | fat: 32.9g | protein: 5.1g | carbs: 50.8g | fiber: 7.0g | sodium: 41mg

www.ingramcontent.com/pod-product-compliance
Lightning Source LLC
Chambersburg PA
CBHW070733030426
42336CB00013B/1963